# Intermittent Fasting for Women

## A Beginner's Guide to Losing Weight Through Intermittent Fasting

# Table of Contents

# Introduction

Back in the 60s and 70s, there wasn't a lot of pressure on people to lose weight. Parents never worried about the excessive weight of their teenage children. Most importantly, people were naturally slim, and life was good. Really good.

But now, things have changed. And dramatically, to say the least. Rather than focusing on losing weight to maintain a healthy lifestyle, people are more worried about fitting into that classy little black dress. More than men, women are obsessed with losing weight, and I can certainly understand why. Apart from being ridiculed for their weight, it's a little more difficult for women to lose weight, and that's when the pressure sets in.

You can lose weight in a variety of ways. Exercising, dieting, etc., but it either takes a long time or it doesn't work at all. Perhaps it's your body type or a genetic problem – and losing weight quickly becomes a losing battle. Most people quit at this point and resign themselves to thinking that it's impossible to lose weight.

Obesity is, indeed, a bigger problem than you think. In fact, it's classified as an epidemic. But, remember that you're not alone. Millions of people struggle day in and day out just like you. According to the WHO, more than 650 million people were obese in 2016! They hate themselves for their inability to lose weight. They give up and simply start binge-eating – something you've probably done many times.

However, there's no need to get so worked up. No matter what the issue is, it can be treated. And, you can do it alone – without anybody's help!

The best way to lose weight is to keep an eye on your diet. But then, you've probably tried many diets that restrict calories, and they haven't worked. From Keto to Atkins to the difficult-to-execute GM diet, you've tried it all. I've tried them too, and I figured that although I lost weight for a while, it came back with a vengeance.

For too many years, we have come to believe that eating foods with less fat or reducing calories will lend a hand in reducing weight. But what if all that is just a misunderstanding? What if I told you that you can lose weight if you treat the cause rather than the symptom? You've probably seen many people lose weight with minimal effort? How does that happen? Well, it's all in the hormones.

To put it simply, it's all about your insulin levels. While other diets make you starve and unhappy, you're also going to gain it back once you stop dieting. However, intermittent fasting is a different beast. It not only makes you shed all those pounds, but you stay that way. Additionally, your focus and energy levels go up too.

So, basically, intermittent fasting works. Don't take my word for it – scientific research backs intermittent fasting. Going back to the tricks of losing weight, the best way to do it is to eat less. As simple as that. However, you don't have to starve yourself. It's all about maintaining a balance, and this book will teach you how to do just that.

# Chapter 1
## Is obesity the main culprit?

Obesity is a slow killer. It may not be alarming in the beginning, but only obese people will understand how deadly it really is. Most doctors suggest going to the gym and exercising. Get fit, they say. Friends ridicule you for not being determined. They say you're lazy and making up excuses for not going to the gym.

When it comes to the diet, they proclaim that you're eating too many carbs. Another doctor will tell you that carbs aren't the problem – they are innocent – but it's the calories you should be worried about. Then, there's another discussion about good and bad carbs and how they affect you, and blah blah.

People will tell you to stay from fried foods – and I agree. You should limit the amount of fried foods you eat. But you begin to wonder – what about people that never lose weight even when they eat healthy food? I'm sure you'll see many examples.

Doctors hand over different types of treatments to their patients and the patients just follow them because they have no other choice. They take advice from even doctors that are obese themselves. If the treatments were so effective, you'd never see an obese doctor in the first place, but I bet you have.

So, what exactly is obesity? It's nothing but an individual's BMI – Body Mass Index – that's calculated using the height and weight of the person. If the BMI exceeds 30, you will be considered an obese person. There are various treatments you'll see to treat obesity including surgery, but with more than 39% of the adult population considered overweight in 2016 alone by WHO, it's nothing short of an epidemic.

Although it's commonly advised to limit calorie intake, that approach hasn't really produced results. Sure, you might lose weight initially, but it usually comes back. On top of that, obesity is associated with many ailments such as diabetes, kidney issues, etc; however, the medications prescribed to cure the disease makes the patient put on more weight. As you can surmise, patients are caught in a vicious circle they can never get out of.

Logically, you'd think that treating obesity is the best method to prevent diseases; however, doctors are more interested in treating the disease rather than paying more attention to obesity itself. Obesity is most often treated as an after-thought rather than the primary issue.

Also, have you noticed that children are obese when their parents also suffer from the same plight? What could be the problem? When some studies note that various factors including behavior, environmental factors, lifestyle, and socio-econic status can lead to obesity, they refuse to take an important factor – genetics – into account.

One of the most important causes of obesity is genetics, and the fact is that you can inherit obesity. This is not to say that you can't reduce weight even if you've inherited obesity. Yes, you can lose weight. However, it's important to determine the cause and treat it rather than blaming environmental factors and lifestyle alone.

Basically, what I want to tell you is that obesity can be treated. If you've tried everything but nothing seems to work, there's no harm in giving intermittent fasting a try.

# Chapter 2
# What is intermittent fasting?

In many countries, fasting is a way of life. People tend to fast during particular time periods according to their religions and belief. For example, Muslims observe a fast during the holy month of Ramadan while Hindus fast during certain festivals. Well, obviously they don't starve for the whole month, but they eat only during specific time frames.

Have you wondered why? For centuries, many people have relied on fasting, and although it hasn't been done to lose weight, the end result is that you shed loads of weight.

Note that I use the word "fast", which is very different than "starve". Right off the bat, you need to understand that fasting and starving are different. While starving leads to muscle loss and various other health issues, fasting ensures that you lose extra weight. Starving isn't planned, but you're in complete control when you're fasting.

Intermittent fasting is nothing but eating food in specific intervals. You simply cycle between periods of eating and fasting. Although many generations have followed intermittent fasting for centuries, most people haven't even heard about it. Thankfully, it's now becoming popular after people have realized that it truly works.

If done right, intermittent fasting can not only cut your weight, but you'll also be able to reverse diseases like diabetes! It sounds far-fetched, but there's a lot of scientific evidence that it actually works. As long as you're not underweight and have reserves of body fat, intermittent fasting is completely safe.

There are many ways to do intermittent fasting, and we will get to that in subsequent chapters. However, you can choose to observe any type of fasting, and it will show results pretty quickly. While some people fast for more than 24 hours, others fast only for 12-18 hours. It totally depends on how committed you are, and most importantly – how your body reacts.

In other words, you will be in complete control and decide how you want to do it. In fact, you may be observing a fast even without your knowledge. For example, if you have your dinner at 7 pm and eat your breakfast at 10 am, you have just fasted for 15 hours! And that's all there is to intermittent fasting.

However, remember that fasting means that you cannot drink coffee with milk or sugar. Or any other sugary drinks for that matter. Sure, black coffee with a couple teaspoons of milk is allowed, but you can't mix in any sugar.

Intermittent fasting is perhaps one of the oldest tricks used to reduce weight. But most people tend to cringe when you mention the word "fast" because they are made to believe that it's good to eat to their heart's content. Eat whatever you want, but make sure you exercise, they say. Some even promote the theory that you must eat at least 5-6 times a day. Yes, the food portions are small but it's not possible for your body to burn fat when you're constantly feeding or overloading it.

All this will become clear when you understand the science behind intermittent fasting. So, let's move on to…

**What's the science behind Intermittent Fasting?**

If you're hearing about IF (Intermittent Fasting, in this case) for the first time, it's easy to discern that you'll lose weight when you skip meals. It's perhaps the same as restricting calories, you think. Right? Wrong.

IF works in a different way. Yes, you eat less than you usually do by skipping one meal, but you'll lose weight more than people that restrict calories. And the best part is that the weight doesn't come back, unlike your usual diets when the weight is back again within a month.

So, how does IF actually work? Well, it works by burning body fat. By restricting food, you're essentially forcing your body to burn fat. This is a practice that has evolved for centuries, so there's nothing new with that.

Understanding how basic principles work will grasp the concept of IF. For that, just think about how people become obese. Lean people also became obese later, so it's not only genetics at play here. But why do they become obese?

Well, it's because the body begins to store excess food as fat. Once you eat, the body derives its energy for normal activities from the food you have consumed. Generally, we ingest more food than necessary, and the excess energy is stored as fat for later use. Insulin – a hormone that plays a key role in our body – helps to store the incoming food as energy.

So, it's easy to understand that body fat is nothing but energy that is stored by the body itself. Since there's excessive energy or food, the fat has nowhere to go. Or, in other words, it doesn't burn, and that's why you have fat deposits in different parts of the body.

Whenever you eat food, insulin supply increases, and although the hormone really helps to store that food to be used as energy later, excessive food leads to a lot of fat that will be stored in different parts.

Insulin actually stores all that excessive food or energy in two ways. The carbohydrates are converted into units of sugar or glucose. The glucose then forms glycogen and is stored in the liver. But since there isn't a lot of space to store the carbs, the liver begins to convert all that excess glucose to fat. And that, ladies and gentlemen, is how body fat is created.

Now, the liver produces body fat, but whatever is in excess is then transported to other parts of the body. These fat deposits simply occur whenever you eat a lot of food and don't give the body a chance to burn it off. And – this is important – since the body can create unlimited fat to use it as energy later, you keep putting on more weight.

The human body has two systems to store energy. First is glycogen and it can be accessed easily. And the second system is the body fat but it's a little difficult to be accessed.

So, now you know what happens when you eat excessively. Or in other terms, you know what happens when you eat more than what your body needs. But what happens if you fast or don't eat for specific periods of time?

The process just reverses. And that's Intermittent Fasting. When you observe IF, the levels of insulin decrease and the body realizes that it needs to burn stored fat as there's no incoming food or energy. To understand this, think of how you spend money.

For example, imagine that you have money in your wallet. You also have some money stored in the bank. If you need to purchase something, you simply use the money that can be accessed immediately. Thus, you first spend money in the wallet, rather than running to the bank every time.

The human body works in a similar fashion. When there's no money in the wallet, you are forced to go the bank to withdraw. Similarly, the body first utilizes glycogen that can be accessed without any difficulty to get energy; however, that energy is sufficient only for the next day or so. Thus, when it runs out of energy and the glucose decreases, it uses the body fat.

It's now easy to understand how the body processes all the fat stores. It's also evident that you're either fasting or eating. You are fasting when you're sleeping, or doing anything other than eating. Or drinking for that matter. Basically, anything that has sugar will be used for energy.

That means that the body has two states where you're either fed or fasting. When you're full, you have a high amount of insulin, and when you've fasted for a while, the insulin slowly drops, and the body is forced to get its energy by decreasing the fat.

To maintain your current body weight, you simply have to make sure that the amount of fat burnt is more than the amount consumed. If the body spends a lot of time in the fed state, it will just store the excess as fat, and it just increases over a period of time. However, if you give your body sufficient time to use its fat, you'll lose weight pretty easily.

And, that is intermittent fasting at its core.

Basically, you're telling your body what to do. Fasting may seem difficult, and even impossible for some people that are used to eating every 3-4 hours; however, it's a very natural thing to do. It may seem difficult in the beginning, but your body is a machine that will adjust easily if you're committed to it.

It's important to convince your mind that there's nothing wrong with IF. Many people will tell you that you're going to fall sick, but it's just not possible unless you're fasting for more than 3-4 days at a time.

If you eat something every 3-4 hours like it's commonly recommended, you're not allowing your body enough time to burn all that energy. But those meals are small, you say. Yes, they may be small portions; however, without a chance to burn that fat, your body has no chance to reduce weight. It's just simple science.

To summarize intermittent fasting in a few words…

IF is a practice that allows your body to maintain a balance between fasting and feasting. Whenever you consume a meal, your body uses it to burn energy. However, when the energy is much more than required, it stores that energy as fat for later use. To burn all that fat or prevent the body from storing fat deposits all over, you must give it some time to process it or burn it. The more time you give, the more fat is burnt. In other words, the more you fast, the more weight you lose.

IF is even more effective if you engage in many activities when you're fasting. Remember how the body uses glycogen as energy? So, if you're working out or doing some strenuous activity in a fasted state, your body will have no choice other than using that stored fat even if it can't be accessed easily.

It works because it's about your sensitivity to insulin. When you're in a fasting state, you are more sensitive to insulin compared to a fed state. This also means that a meal after a workout will help the body use the energy in an efficient manner since the glycogen that's entering your body will be used as energy immediately. Since there's no extra energy, the body will not store it as fat.

Through IF, you're simply teaching your body a better way to use the food. Rather than storing it, it learns to burn the fat and use it as fuel to do any activity. By depriving your body of new calories, you're simply burning fat. As simple as that!

All this is fine and dandy, but is there any difference when it comes to women? Do women react differently when they observe IF?

# Chapter 3
# Is intermittent fasting different for women?

Thanks to all the myths surrounding IF, it becomes difficult to believe anything. And it makes it especially confusing when physicians tell you that you'll actually increase weight when you fast. It's incredible that people actually believe that missing a single meal can result in serious diseases.

Some people I know are so paranoid about missing meals that they impose their opinions on others. And believe it or not, it's made even more difficult for women. Even if you somehow believe in the benefits of fasting, you are told that it affects women in a different way.

You've probably read articles on how IF can make women infertile! That's not only ridiculous, but it's like saying that women who have fasted for several days and even months all these years are infertile.

Of course, women shouldn't fast when they are pregnant, but that goes without saying. The same goes for women that are underweight. Why would you even want to fast and lose weight if you're underweight anyway? Much of what is said about IF doesn't make sense, but it is insane to make women believe that IF isn't effective only for them. Somehow, you're led to understand that while IF may work for men, it's a total waste for women.

Well, it's time to set the record straight. Hell, that's why I decided to write this book! I believe that IF works not only for men, but it's amazing even for women. Just ask all those Buddhist, Hindu and Muslim women that have fasted for religious purposes. Really, it doesn't affect you adversely at all.

Just before we proceed, however, I want to make it entirely clear that pregnant women shouldn't be fasting. I said that earlier, but it needs to repeated. Children shouldn't fast either. No religion allows that anyway. And it makes total sense because children and pregnant women need all the nutrition they can get.

If you're pregnant, you should be looking for ways to get as much nutrition as possible by eating fresh food, so IF will not work. Moreover, why would you try to diet or lose weight when you're pregnant anyway? It's simply going against nature, and it won't work.

Yes, women do face a few issues while fasting. For example, some women find it incredibly difficult to suppress their hunger pangs, but the same applies for men too. Yes, women also have difficulties reducing weight quickly, but men also have the same problem. There's no difference really.

In fact, women have a higher threshold compared to men when it comes to pain. Your body is such a superior machine that it withstands pain. Thus, fasting shouldn't be an issue. Like all diets, you simply get used to it.

Still, I understand that you have doubts. Can it affect my metabolism? Will I have problems if I want to bear children?

What if I'm already a mother? These are probably some of the questions you're asking right now. So, let's take a good look at the facts.

Women – just like men – have a long history of fasting. Your metabolism will not be affected even if you fast for a week while eating during specific periods of time. Again, I want to reiterate that IF is not a process where you fast for days together. You pick time periods where you're comfortable eating or comfortable fasting. It's intermittent. And, like men, women will have no problems.

Doctors have prescribed IF as an effective and safe way to reduce weight without any dire medical consequences. For instance, Dr. Gilliland published a study where 46 patients were told to fast for 14 days! That's almost a fortnight. Interestingly, 32 individuals were females and they faced no issues whatsoever. Still, you see many articles telling you that fasting is a complete no-no.

Of course, you see advertisements and even TV shows featuring "experts" telling you that fasting is detrimental. A friend of mine tells me that fasting will lead to liver and kidney failure. I don't even know what to say to that because when you're in complete denial, nothing can be done.

So, what were the results of the study conducted by Dr. Gilliland, you ask? First off, 44 patients completed the fasting process without a hitch. While one individual decided to quit, another developed nausea. However, 44 people successfully completed a 2-week fast! While some think that it's difficult to skip a meal, you can see that it's really not impossible.

The patients were allowed to drink tea, sugarless coffee, and water during those 14 days. On average, they lost about 17.2 pounds or 8 kilos in that period. After they were discharged, all the participants were asked to follow a low-calorie diet that exceeded no more than 600 to 1000 calories.

Some participants even asked to re-enter the program! The three diabetic patients successfully stopped their insulin medications at the end of the fast and others achieved similarly positive results. Another important information you must note is that the participants gained some of their lost weight back after they returned to their regular lives. Why? Well, it's because of the fact that the weight they lost initially was primarily water.

As soon as they began to eat normally, some of the weight was regained; however, they successfully shed most of their weight. This may happen to you initially too. The weight you lose at the very beginning will be back once you start eating normally. However, you will be able to lose most of the fat, and it won't come back. You also will feel better and sharper, thanks to IF. Contrary to what people say, fasting actually resets your body and enables you to perform better.

The participants also noted that while the fasting was successful for them, the low-calorie restrictions didn't work for them later. It's also important to note that most individuals didn't bother to follow the diet after they finished the fasting program.

At the end of it all, it's scientifically proven that fasting can and will help you lose weight. Many of the participants were women. So, yeah, it works for women too. There's no question about that. In fact, it may work much better for women than men.

It's natural to live life in cycles. Sometimes you feast during special occasions. And, sometimes you need to fast when you have too much fat stored in the body. If you successfully maintain this intermittent balance, you will be able to lead a better life.

If anything, the difference between fasting for men and women is that the plasma glucose levels tend to reduce faster for women. Plasma glucose test or FPG is a method used to test the blood sugar levels of patients after they have fasted for at least 8 hours.

In addition, women also experience a state of ketosis much faster than men. Ketosis is a very natural process that occurs in the human body when there's a dearth of carbs. Generally, carbs are burned as fuel for energy but when the body is low on carbs, it burns fat instead and produces ketones, which is known as ketosis.

However, the differences reduce as time goes on. Also, there isn't a lot of difference in the amount of weight both men and women lose. At the end of the day, fasting is almost the same for both the genders.

# Chapter 4
## Types of intermittent fasting

There are different ways to do intermittent fasting. Honestly, that's the best part about it. If you're worried about fasting for an entire day, there are different approaches and you can do something that suits you.

Due to its popularity, there are many different versions, but I suggest you keep it simple. Remember, IF is nothing but a state where you're sometimes feasting and fasting at other times. Intermittently. Also, note that any method will work, as long as you stick to it. I just want to reiterate again that any of these iterations will suit women. If you're concerned about fasting as a woman, read chapter 3 again!

So, let's a look at the different ways of practicing IF.

### 1) Fast only for 1 or 2 days per week

IF may seem intimidating at first, but it becomes very easy once you get used to it. However, you may need some help to get used to it. As a beginner, it makes sense to choose something that's easier rather than waging a battle from the very first day.

Some people begin fasting every alternate day as soon as they start IF, but it's not necessary. Start by indulging in a fast that lasts for a day or 24 hours, and see how you feel. Brad Pilon – a fitness expert – popularized this method, and many people seem to follow it.

So, if you eat dinner today at 8 pm, for instance, make sure you eat nothing until 8 pm the next day. Hey, I get that you're a busy lady and you're probably feeling uncomfortable to go to work without eating breakfast. But, don't worry, you'll be surprised by how quickly your body adjusts to it.

If you can't imagine skipping breakfast, try eating breakfast, but the catch is that you can't eat until breakfast the next day. Whatever you do, you have to fast for 24 hours. Of course, you need to drink loads of water during the fasting period. Also, coffee and tea are allowed, but you cannot use sugar.

Imagine you start with the 24-hour fast and find yourself ravenous as you reach the 16-hour mark. What do you do? You simply adjust. There's another method for you as well.

## 2) 16/8 Intermittent fasting

As the name suggests, you've probably understood by now that the 16/8 fast indicates that you fast for 16 hours a day. However, the catch is that you have to do this every day, or it won't work.

Let's imagine you eat breakfast at 8 am. You cannot have anything in between except coffee, tea and water until it's 12 am. Obviously, this is not going to work for many people. So, you can adjust the timing a bit. Or, you can have dinner at 8 pm and have lunch at 12 pm the next day. Whatever your choice, make sure you fast for at least 15-16 hours.

Unlike other types of intermittent fasting, the 16/8 fast dictates that you keep up with this routine every day. Also known as Leangains protocol, this method is very popular among those that can't stand 24-hour fasts. By eating dinner and only skipping breakfast, you've got a window of 16 hours that includes the time you sleep!

Let me tell you that most women start their intermittent fasting journey through this method. Why? Well, it's because it's ridiculously easy and requires you to skip a single meal – breakfast – for you to enjoy the benefits of the fast.

Those that avoid eating breakfast on a regular basis will enjoy this version of IF. Another thing you need to remember that is you can't indulge in junk food. You can't fast for 16 hours and gorge on burgers and fries during the 8-hour window. I mean, why would you? It doesn't make sense to put in all that effort and let it all go to waste.

So, if you can't do the 24-hour fast once or twice a week, start with the 16/8 fast and you'll see that it's not all that difficult.

## 3) 5:2 Intermittent Fasting

The 5:2 is very similar to the first version of IF described above. However, the difference is that you're not going to actually fast on any day. Instead of fasting that requires you to not eat anything at all, you simply restrict calories for only two days a week while you eat regular food on the remaining 5 days of the week.

Made popular by a doctor named Michael Mosley, this diet is very popular among those that don't want to fast. According to the 5:2 diet, you can consume only up to 500 calories if you're a woman and 600 calories for men. Of course, it's 500 calories per day and not 500 calories for 5 days, just in case you're wondering how you're going to survive!

So, for instance, if you decide to "fast" on Monday and Wednesday, you only eat up to 500 calories on those two days. However, you can eat regular food during the other days. As you can understand by now, this type of diet is a little different because you're not technically fasting at all. However, by restricting calories, you will see the difference in your body weight soon. It's not as good as the other types of IF, but you can certainly start with the 5:2 diet if you find it impossible to fast from the very first day.

## 4) Feast and Fast

IF is all about putting your body through a stage of feasting and fasting. So, I can hear some of you thinking, "Can I feast during the day and fast at night?" Or, can you fast during the day and feast at night? Yep, you can.

Popularized as "Warrior Diet" by a fitness expert named Ori Hofmekler, this diet involves eating a bit and then fasting. In other words, you're feasting as well as fasting. However, the term "fasting" is wrong here, because you're not really fasting. Instead, you're restricting calories by eating unprocessed, whole foods.

Simply put, you're going to have to eat fruits or vegetables during the day. At night, you can whatever you want. Technically, you're going to reduce calories and force your body to reduce weight.

## 5)  Skip meals whenever possible

Some people cannot adjust to a set routine. No matter how hard they try, they find it difficult to fast. Whether it's hectic schedule or kids making you run around all day, some women find it impossible to carry on without eating anything.

If that's you, you can simply skip meals whenever possible. For instance, if you're too bored to cook for yourself, simply skip that particular meal. Let's say you haven't eaten anything this afternoon. If you eat at night, you are indeed practicing IF because you've skipped a meal.

Don't worry about people telling you that it isn't healthy to skip meals. Honestly, you're doing your body a favor. Even if you're in your 30s or 40s, skipping a meal does not hurt. Of course, there are many people – even doctors – that will tell you to eat small meals at regular intervals. But, if you want to lose weight, IF is the way to go. Also, remember to eat healthier meals whenever you skip the previous meal to help your body gain as much nutrition as possible.

## 6)  Fasting every alternate day

Once you've tried other fasting methods mentioned above, you may be keen to try fasting every alternate day. Or maybe not. Depends on how it works for you. But, whatever your reason, make sure you try fasting every alternate day at least for 1 week to truly gain the benefits of IF.

Honestly, fasting every alternate day is not as brutal as you think because you're not technically fasting. This is because you're allowed to eat during the fasting period, but you must ensure that you restrict calories.

So, for instance, if you're fasting on Monday, you're allowed to eat up to 500 calories. On Tuesday, though, you can eat whatever you want, provided it's not junk food.

## The big question – Which version works the best?

Yes, that's a good question. Out of all the versions, there must be something that works better than the rest. You can skip meals, feast and fast, and still not get results as fast as you wish. And, that's because you're providing immediate energy in the form of glycogen your body uses. According to IF, your body starts burning fat when you deprive it of glycogen.

Thus, the version that actually works is the 16/8 fast where you eat only within an 8-hour window. However, this can be irritating to some people – including me – where you do it every single day of the week.

I need something I can get it over with. Rather than fasting for 16 hours every day, I find that fasting for once or twice a week works the best for me. I took it to the next level by fasting every alternate day once I was sure that my body had adjusted to it. Similarly, you can try skipping meals randomly and then hop on a regime that actually works for you.

Obviously, you will not see quick changes at the beginning, but if you actually fast for 24 hours for at least two days a week and continue doing so for several months at least, you will see results.

# Chapter 5
# Reducing body set weight

According to dietary studies, almost all diets fail over a period of time. Whether you restrict calories, fat, or carbs, you will regain all the weight you lost with a vengeance. Don't you remember giving up after trying a new diet? It's the same with everyone else. Atkins, GM diet, Paleo – no matter what, the weight comes back.

Have you wondered why?

Well, it's because of the way the human body is designed. Like everything else, weight loss also follows a pattern. And you can relate to this. Sure, you lose weight as soon as you start a new diet. You continue losing weight for maybe 5-6 months, but what happens after that? Your body resists weight loss and you regain all that weight.

This particular occurrence, known as weight-loss plateau, is very common. It also occurs because your body sets a particular weight, and soon as you cross the threshold, it resists losing more weight. A very famous physician – Dr. Jason Fung – who actively supports Intermittent Fasting – refers to this as a thermostat where the temperature is already set.

Dr Rudolph Leibel was the physician who proved that the body works like a thermostat. Now, what exactly does that mean? Dr Jason Fung explains this clearly. Let's imagine that you've set the thermostat regulating the temperature of your house to 50°F

(10°C) instead of the usual 70°F or 21°C. Most people would find this environment cold.

Normally, you'd adjust the thermostat; however, if you decide to reduce the temperature through other means, you'd purchase a heater. At first, the temperature increases due to the heater; however, the thermostat springs into action as soon as the temperature exceeds the set condition and switches on the air conditioner.

Now, what you have on your hands is a battle between the air conditioner and the heater where both are struggling against each other. At the end of the day, the thermostat does everything to make the temperature go back to its set condition – i.e. 50°F (10°C).

The mistake here lies in the fact that instead of adjusting the temperature of the thermostat (changing the set temperature) to reduce the cold, we buy a heater to counter the problem. Similarly, we fight against our very own body to reduce weight, and that's the core of the problem.

Like the thermostat, out body also sets a weight. No matter what you do, it fights against you to manage that particular weight. And it works both ways. Just like it's hard to reduce weight, it's hard to increase weight.

Coming back to Dr Rudolph Leibel, he proved this concept by testing his theory on a group of 10 people. At first, the individuals were overfed to make them increase weight. Then, their food intake was reduced, and they lost weight. Remarkably, it was observed that as the individuals put on weight, the energy expenditure of their bodies also increased proportionally. Likewise, as they reduced weight, the energy expenditure slowed down to counter weight-loss.

As you can understand by now, the human body adjusts itself to meet the set condition – like a thermostat. This also explains why it's so hard to lose all that fat! As soon as you start reducing weight, the body actively resists it by slowing your metabolism. If you put on weight, it increases the metabolism in an effort to lose that weight. It's like fighting against your own self to achieve something!

And this also explains why most diets fail. As soon as you lose a certain amount of weight, the body thermostat kicks in and you hit the dreaded weight plateau – a point where you no longer reduce weight, and all the lost weight comes back again.

So, what's the solution here, you ask? Well, just like you can solve the problem by adjusting the temperature of the thermostat instead of getting a new heater, you can adjust the set weight of your body so that the weight you've lost doesn't come back again.

Obese people find it particularly hard to lose weight because the body metabolism slows down and their appetite also increases – two conditions that make it super difficult for them to lose weight. Instead of treating the problem, we need to focus on treating the cause.

For instance, think of why we become obese. Is it the calories? Or sleep deprivation? Or is it the insulin resistance? The truth is that they all cause obesity, which means that it's not one single reason that causes obesity. Since there are many factors involved, we need to understand how they work to treat obesity, rather than focusing on just calories or sugar.

Also, many types of diets work, depending on how your body reacts to it. You don't need to choose one side. Low-carb diet, low-fat diet, low-calorie diet – they all work, but only for a while. Ultimately, you just gain all the weight back. I'm sure many dieters will relate to this, because sometimes you feel like no matter how hard you try, you simply fail.

Having said that, the best to attack weight gain is to keep an eye on the insulin levels. Why? Just recall that obesity doesn't occur due to calories. Instead, it's a result of hormonal imbalance. The insulin present in our body dictates it to start storing all the food we eat as fat. But, when the levels of insulin go down, some of that fat quickly burns off. This also explains why we simply don't fall dead whenever we fast!

Remember how the reference of a thermostat was used to compare it with the Body Set Weight or BSW? If the temperature is too high, the thermostat springs into action until the temperature returns back to normal. Similarly, the human body also utilizes the same theory. Whenever there's excess insulin, the fat cells increase.

To counter this, the body produces a hormone known as leptin that signals to the brain that we are putting on weight. As soon as the brain receives this message, we stop eating because the appetite decreases quickly. At this point, the insulin also decreases and the body takes this as an indication to burn excess fat and to stop consuming any food.

As you can see, BSW works on a feedback loop, which goes something like this:

High Insulin → Gain weight → Leptin increases → Appetite decreases → Insulin reduces → eat again and increase insulin. And the process just repeats. (To understand more about insulin, refer to Chapter 7).

As you can see, the human body is a very complex and balanced system that doesn't let you become too fat or too thin. Just like it's difficult to lose weight, it's very tough to gain weight. And, this is also why you can't eat more than your capacity. Ever tried to eat more than 10 pounds of chicken at a time? Nope? It's because it's not possible, all thanks to your body's mechanism.

The loop shown above works to keep your body weight stable despite the havoc we create by eating too much. But, if that's the case, how does one become obese, you ask? Well, obesity is a slow process. It takes time, and the weight keeps increasing little by little whenever we abuse our bodies by stuffing our faces with cookies, cakes, etc. The reverse is also true because you can reduce your weight a little every time by fasting and maintaining a sugar-free diet whenever possible.

You can display a higher insulin level due to several factors including sleep deprivation, excessive intake of sugar, and more. Thus, understanding why your insulin levels are so high will help you reduce weight and also reduce the set body weight at the same time. In other words, if you lower the set body weight, you will not be fighting against yourself to lose weight.

As higher insulin levels are the culprit that makes you gain weight, it makes sense to target insulin and lower its levels. But, how can you actually do that? Well, there are many ways.

# Chapter 6
# Focus on what to eat

So, since insulin is such a big contributor in increasing weight, you can reduce insulin levels by concentrating on what you eat. And, this is how you reduce your body set weight. Here are a few ways to do that...

## 1) Stop snacking unnecessarily

Nowadays, you have all sorts of experts telling you to eat at least 6 meals a day. Of course, they tell you to eat smaller proportions, but do you think it really matters? Even in the 60s, people were accustomed to eating only 3 meals a day. Obesity was never a problem in the past like it is today. They even had access to a lot of snacks. Most importantly, they loved white bread that was loaded with sugar. So, what exactly changed?

Well, it's because of the timing. As you already know, intermittent fasting is a state where your body is sometimes in a feast mode and sometimes in the fast mode. Earlier, although people used to consume about 3 meals a day, they didn't eat a lot of snacks like we do today. We are told to eat about 6 meals a day, so you imagine what that does to the body where it doesn't even have time to spend the energy you've just consumed.

In the past, people ate food in such a way that there was a considerable difference between periods of high and low insulin levels. Or fast and feast modes. Since they spent a good amount of time fasting (due to eating only 3 meals a day) their bodies never had the problem of insulin resistance that makes it hard to lose weight. Obesity didn't have a huge chance to develop because they spent a good amount of time with low insulin levels.

Similarly, you can keep your insulin in check by reducing snacks. In fact, it's best to not snack at all. It does sound horrific because you're no longer going to be able to eat chips or cookies whenever you feel like, but if you want to reduce insulin and decrease your body set weight, you need to follow the rules.

Snacks contain a great amount of sugar and refined flour that raise insulin levels. Muffins, hot-dogs, cookies, jellies, biscuits, and other calorie-rich snacks will make you put on weight! So, what do you do? You stop snacking. At least for now, because you need to reduce that set weight. If you cannot control the urge to snack, replace your snacks with something healthier – like whole foods that are in season.

## 2) Stop eating dessert after every meal

There are many people – including myself – who cannot resist a big dessert after a big meal. In fact, we continue eating desserts to such an extent that it becomes an important part of our daily diet. Guess what that does? Yep, it makes you put on weight relentlessly. So, what's the solution? Simple – stop eating desserts.

Desserts are nothing but sugars disguised as something else. They look so tasty that you just cannot help yourself. Whether you love cakes, cookies, ice cream or whatever melts your heart, they ultimately raise your insulin levels, making it a lot harder to reduce weight.

Candies are the biggest culprits because they are nothing but small balls of sugar coated with a fragrant and tasty flavor. As soon as you make it a habit to eat desserts every time you finish a meal, you're losing the battle right there.

Thus, replacing desserts with healthier alternatives like nuts and seasonal fruits is a good way to keep your weight in check. Rather than eating that candy that doesn't contribute in any way to a healthier lifestyle, eating a bowl of nuts and cherries will serve you better. Even dark chocolate that mostly contains cacao instead of sugar is a better option. However, stay away from white chocolate or any chocolate that's processed with just sugar.

Basically, remember that you cannot indulge in eating desserts every day. Of course, there will be occasions where you can't avoid snacking on desserts – and that's okay – but try not to do it frequently so that it keeps your insulin levels in check.

## 3) Do not consume sugar

Sugar is the biggest culprit in increasing weight. Guess why? Yes, it's because it works fast and hard to stimulate insulin secretion. The sad part of eating sugar is that it doesn't even work temporarily – it works to increase insulin in the long term.

Sugar contains both fructose and glucose, and they contribute to insulin resistance in a wonderful manner. If you're resistant to insulin for a longer period, you ultimately have higher levels of insulin that makes you put on weight relentlessly.

In simple terms, sugar makes you fat. Much fatter than you can imagine. And, the horrible part is that there's no physical limit to eating sugar. You can eat more than 20 candies in a day and you won't bat an eyelid. You can also polish off an entire tub of ice-cream without any resistance from your body. Sad part is that you won't feel the effects immediately but the long term effects are what you should be concerned about. Sugar directly works on increasing insulin resistance, and it has zero nutritional benefits.

Thus, the solution here is to eliminate added sugar. Note that the keyword here is "added sugar" because you'll find sugar even in natural foods. Any type of fruit will have sugar but that's not the same as added sugar. What differs is the concentration and amount of sugar. For example, eating an orange is not the same as eating a teaspoon of sugar. You cannot avoid eating natural foods. Therefore, your best bet is to avoid commercially prepared snacks with a lot of sugar.

But, how do I know if packaged food contains sugar, you ask? Well, you don't, and that's part of the problem. To avoid eating foods with sugar, you have to pay close attention to the labels. Manufacturers use various other names to conceal the real ingredient. And, that's why you see pseudonyms like glucose, sucrose, fructose, etc.

Commercial foods contain high amounts of sugar, but that doesn't mean all natural foods are okay. Honey, for instance, is basically sugar although it's natural. It's the same if you consume 6-8 oranges or a tall glass of orange juice in one sitting. Even foods like plain white bread, jams, jellies, peanut butter, etc. contain sugar. Fruits contain fructose that aids in weight-gain, so it's best to eat them in moderation. However, natural foods don't contain as much sugar as commercial foods.

To put it simply, remember that everything natural isn't necessarily great for the body, especially when it contains sugar in any form.

To avoid sugar, stay away from commercial foods like sauces and syrups. Syrups, in particular, contain a heavy amount of sugar. Sugar is added to sauces also to enhance the flavor. Basically, your best bet is to stick to fruits that are sweet if you crave for it, but even that should be moderated.

## 4) Drink healthy beverages

Honestly, there aren't many options when it comes to beverages when you're fasting because almost every beverage is loaded with sugar. As long as there's no sugar, you can drink pretty much anything. However, drinks like fruit juice, soda, milk shakes, smoothies, and similar drinks are a big no-no.

The best way to work around this problem is make the drink yourself. For instance, coffee is a wonderful option because not only does it contain a great number of antioxidants, but it also aids in weight-loss. Adding a couple teaspoons of milk is okay if you cannot stand black coffee. You can also add hot chocolate (dark chocolate that contains no sugar) to your regular coffee to make it more enjoyable.

Iced coffee is also an amazing way to get rid of your hunger when you're fasting. Adding extracts like vanilla will improve the taste and reduce your hunger pangs to a great extent. Of course, your iced coffee shouldn't contain any milk or cream because...well, that's sugar again.

The same applies to tea. Green tea is very popular. In fact, there are many different types of teas that help you improve your focus and make the fasting a lot more bearable. You could also make iced tea, but make sure that the iced tea powder you use doesn't have any sugar in it.

Some diets allow you to drink alcohol in moderate amounts, but you cannot touch alcohol if you're fasting. And that's because alcohol is nothing but fermented sugar. While beer is fermented barley, other hard drinks like vodka and whiskey also contain excessive amounts of sugar.

The best part of observing Intermittent Fasting is that it's mandatory to drink lots of water. Not only does it make your skin clearer, but drinking a lot of water frequently also helps you reduce a lot of weight. You will notice that it becomes easy to shed fat if you depend on water.

You can also add small amounts of apple cider vinegar to your water to make it tastier. Or, use lemon juice. However, it's not the same as a lemonade you'd get in a cafe, for instance. Lemonades, just like other beverages such as milk shakes and smoothies, also contain sugar.

**Important note** – You may be tempted to add artificial sweeteners, especially the ones that are advertised as sugar-free. However, artificial sweeteners also have sucrose or sugar in another form. It's the same at the end of the day, so artificial sweeteners don't work. The same applies to natural sweeteners like honey or agave syrup.

Even maple syrup, for that matter. No matter how natural they are, they will add sugar to your diet and all your hard work will ultimately be wasted. Therefore, don't add any type of sugar to your beverages – natural or commercial. The human body doesn't distinguish between natural or processed sugar, which makes it really hard to lose weight even if you're fasting.

## 5) Skip breakfast or any meal if you aren't hungry

This is already mentioned in "Types of Intermittent Fasting". But I am reiterating it again because it's the best way to start off with IF if you're a beginner. If fasting intimidates you, start off by skipping any meal.

You've been told that breakfast is something you should never miss. In fact, many doctors will tell that you simply can't skip breakfast or you'll pay heavily for it later. However, this is just not true. Breakfast – as the name suggests – is a meal that allows you to "break" your "fast" just after you wake up.

Notice that the keyword is that you should just break the fast. You can break your fast by consuming something light; however, many people in the breakfast fad to such an extent that they make it the most critical meal of the day. Rather than starting the day by eating something light, we indulge in croissants, donuts topped with chocolate glaze and cream, and other sugar-laden foods.

If you cannot imagine skipping breakfast, go ahead and dig into your meal, but make sure that it's a healthy one. There's no reason to eat a greasy or sugary meal, especially when it's the first meal of your day.

The biggest problem with eating a healthy breakfast is that commercial breakfast foods are nothing but processed foods with lots of sugar and very little nutrition. Breakfast cereals boast of a lot more sugar than you can imagine. Even the foods you get for your children are stuffed with sugar, so be careful and read the labels if you want to avoid sugar.

After all this, you're probably wondering how you're even going to survive! I know, I thought the same. With restriction on everything sweet, there's no way you can even think of doing IF if you have a sweet-tooth. However, it's not that bad. Remember that you can eat anything, but do it moderation. Drinking too much water can also be dangerous at times. And the same rule applies to all the junk food and sweets you eat.

The best way to start IF is to begin with the 16:8 diet. Later, once your body adjusts to it, you can start fasting for 1-3 days every week. Women find it best to fast for 2 days alternatively. For instance, if you fast on Monday, you can skip fasting on Tuesday and fast again on Wednesday.

# Chapter 7
# What causes obesity

There are several causes for obesity, but the most obvious one is insulin. Here's how insulin works:

## Insulin

Insulin is a very important hormone without which the body cannot process sugar. Released by the pancreas, it encourages the human system to utilize the glucose or sugar derived from carbohydrates. Where do the carbohydrates come from? They come from the food we ingest. Insulin helps the body use the sugar so that it has the required energy to perform any activity.

The cells of the human system need glucose for energy. Once you eat food, there's a fresh supply of energy in the form of sugar. But, there's one problem – the sugar doesn't have the ability to enter the cells directly. Thus, as soon as you consume food and the levels of blood sugar increases, the beta cells (cells in the pancreas) receive a signal to release insulin into the bloodstream.

At this point, insulin attaches itself to the cells and also sends signals to absorb the sugar present in the bloodstream. As you can surmise, the body cannot use sugar derived from food without the assistance of insulin. Therefore, it's often referred to as the key hormone that unlocks cells and allows sugar to be utilized properly as energy.

Insulin works in a very sophisticated way. If there's more sugar than required present in the body, it helps you store it in the liver.

The stored sugar is released when the levels of blood sugar are low. It also releases it when you engage in any physical activity or between meals. Insulin works like a balancing scale to keep your blood sugar levels normal. If the levels increase in any case, the pancreas takes care of the problem by secreting more insulin.

It's obvious now that the body cannot function normally without the presence of insulin. When there's less insulin because the body isn't producing much of it, or even if the cells develop a resistance to insulin, you will suffer from high blood sugar or hyperglycemia. Those suffering from type 1 diabetes will be familiar with this situation. To counter this, doctors prescribe insulin injections to process the glucose.

While people suffering from type 1 diabetes have the inability to create insulin, victims of type 2 diabetes don't respond to insulin. In other words, they display a resistance to insulin. For this reason, they take insulin shots to process sugar.

Without insulin, the body cannot even access sugar, and that's exactly why it's so important. But the biggest drawback is that it can make you or anyone fat. Regardless of how much you exercise, spend time in the gym working out, cut down on the calories and carbs – no matter what you do, insulin can make you obese.

It doesn't happen overnight. Nobody becomes obese all of a sudden. It creeps up on you. The jeans you wore last year is a little too tight today. That little black dress you wore after a 3-month diet? Forget about it. Because it doesn't fit you anymore. Before you realize it, you're obese, and then you spend lots of time wondering how to cut weight. That's how insulin works.

There's <u>scientific evidence</u> that excess insulin can lead to weight gain. Obese people struggle with high levels of insulin secretion over a period of time. Compared to people with a normal weight, their insulin levels are high. The levels of insulin strangely have an effect even on waist circumference, sadly. How does insulin behave with lean people? Well, their insulin levels return to normal pretty quickly compared to obese people.

If you've ever tried to measure the amount of insulin present, you'll realize that it's a hard task because it doesn't remain constant throughout. Depending on the type of food you ingest, it fluctuates randomly. However, it's possible to calculate an average figure by constantly measuring the levels all through the day. It's also easier to measure insulin after a fasting period – i.e. right after you wake up.

Many people question whether high insulin actually leads to obesity. Forget scientific evidence for a minute because it can be easily proved without lab reports. People that are given insulin injections become obese over a period of time. That in itself is proof that insulin does have a close relationship with obesity. Fact is that the more insulin you take, the more obese you become.

Insulin is used to treat both type 1 and type 2 diabetes. Although those with type 1 need insulin injections because they lack insulin, patients with type 2 diabetes display high insulin levels and are resistant to it. Sometimes, they are treated with the help of a few oral medications including Metformin, Sulfonylureas, and Meglitinides.

In one particular <u>study</u>, scientists compared a high insulin dose with a standard dose in order to control blood glucose for those suffering from type 1 diabetes. The patients were analyzed after 6 years and the results showed that the patients had fewer complications just because the blood sugar was controlled.

But there was a problem. The participants no doubt enjoyed their relatively healthier lives, but they had gained a lot more weight than before. With a weight gain of 4.5 kilos or 9.8 pounds, the participants had put on more weight than they normally did. Before the trial, both the groups that were studied were not obese. However, since there was a great difference in the levels of insulin they were administered with, they had gained weight.

There are many more studies that highlight weight gain especially after a dose of insulin. Some medications used to treat patients also contain insulin. As you can understand now, you don't gain weight immediately. Instead, it occurs over a period of time. And that's exactly what insulin medications do.

Whether you administer insulin through medications or injections, the result is the same. How do we know? Well, scientists have even tested if there's a difference in weight gain due to the way the patient takes insulin. According to a study conducted in 2007, scientists compared 3 ways of administering insulin. The results showed that all the three protocols made participants gain weight. However, those with high insulin doses gained far more weight than those administered with low doses.

But what happens if you take insulin and reduce eating at the same time, you ask? Amazing idea, eh? Nope that doesn't work either. Take this <u>study</u> into consideration. Researchers used high doses of insulin to normalize blood sugar levels on a group of participants suffering from type 2 diabetes. The test ran for over 6 months where insulin doses were increased slowly every day.

On the other hand, the participants also reduced their caloric intake by about 300 calories. The results showed that while the levels of blood sugar were satisfying, the patients put on at least 8.7 kilos or 19 pounds in weight! By now, it was obvious that insulin increased weight even if the patient reduced calories. Additionally, insulin makes you gain weight even if you don't have diabetes.

Based on all the evidence, it's natural to wonder that if insulin makes you increase weight, the opposite must be true? In other words, would you lose weight if you reduced insulin somehow? And, the answer is: yes, you definitely lose weight if you reduced insulin.

Think about type 1 diabetes, for instance. You already know that it's a disease that makes the pancreas weak by destroying its ability to produce insulin. When you have type 1 diabetes, the levels of insulin fall to extremely low levels.

But have you noticed how patients lose weight drastically? No matter what or how much the patient eats, he or she cannot put on weight. In fact, type 1 diabetes was so dangerous that it was fatal. One fine day, Frederick G Banting discovered insulin, and so many people could breathe a sigh of relief.

Today, patients are injected with insulin and although it helps to cure the disorder, it makes them put on weight. I know you're thinking that since the best way to lose weight is to reduce insulin, why not do that instead of fasting, right? Wrong. Many have probably pondered on this, and that's how a condition known as diabulimia was detected.

Diabulimia is a condition where people deliberately reduce insulin to lose weight for cosmetic purposes. Although it sounds amazing, it's super dangerous. Thus, it's best to focus on fasting and reduce your BSW rather than doing things that may affect your health in the long term.

The theory of whether insulin increases weight has been tested through various medications as well. Not surprisingly, medications that increase insulin cause weight gain while those that reduce insulin levels cause weight loss. Medications that don't affect insulin levels don't exhibit any difference in weight at all.

Take this study into consideration. It concludes that about 75% of weight loss mechanisms in obesity can be predicted just with the levels of insulin. It's not about the calories or not exercising enough. It's simply all about insulin. Eventually, as the insulin keeps increasing, your BSW or Body Set Weight also increases because the body receives signals from the hypothalamus to increase weight.

In simple words, you feel hungry and then eat something. Even if you restrict calories or choose to eat food that has 0 calories (which is pretty tough) your body's energy expenditure decreases and you gain weight regardless. It's an uphill battle to reduce weight. You're stuck in a vicious cycle again.

It's simple to understand that you don't become fat due to overeating. On the contrary, you overeat because you are fat already. But why are we obese? Well, it's because the BSW levels are so high that it becomes almost impossible to lose any weight. But why is the BSW high? The answer lies in insulin.

It's evident that insulin makes you put on weight. Due to the food we eat, insulin increases. But there's another factor that increases the levels of insulin, and it occurs over a period of time. What might that be? Well, it's insulin resistance.

## Insulin resistance

Insulin resistance is responsible for many diseases including Alzheimer's, cancer, heart disease, and more. But what is it exactly? I'll explain.

You are already familiar with the role of insulin. It's a hormone that regulates the levels of blood sugar and does its best to keep them in a normal range. Every time you eat something, blood sugar increases and the pancreas produces more insulin. All this is fine, but what happens when the levels of insulin become way too high?

Think about it. Insulin works like a treasurer that stores fat. It does not like it when the stored fat in the body is broken down to be used as energy. It also encourages the fat cells in the body to stock fat. However, note that insulin is detected during periods of high blood sugar. And, that happens just after you consume a meal.

The body, at this point of experiencing high levels of blood sugar, will not break down the fat stores because it already has surplus energy. Think of it this way – you're running a business. You get your inventory and wait for the sales. Now, you will purchase new stock only when your inventory depletes, isn't it? Why would you purchase more when you already have products in surplus? Doesn't make sense, right?

That's how the body performs too. When there's excess glucose, the body begins to store all that fat, and insulin works hard and tells cells to store it. The pancreas keeps producing insulin. But eventually there comes a point when the cells have had enough of it. Like they say, too much is too bad, and the cells also become unresponsive to insulin.

Does the pancreas recognize the problem and stop producing insulin? No, it doesn't work like that. Instead, it keeps producing more and more insulin as you keep eating more. However, there's a huge problem now that the insulin receptors present in cells stop responding to excess insulin. This is what is called insulin resistance.

This is how you develop hyperinsulinemia where there's excess insulin. One also develops hyperglycemia due to high blood sugar. It's kind of obvious that it's almost impossible to burn any fat at this point. This is because you have too much energy and the body doesn't have a chance to even break it down. This leads to the individual becoming heavier or obese.

Other than contributing to obesity, a lot more happens when insulin increases in the body. Stress hormones are released, signaling that the body must prepare for a stressful environment.

From blood pressure to the heart rate, a lot goes haywire. Stress hormones attack the immune system and also elevate cholesterol in the bloodstream. This is also why you find it difficult to sleep at times when insulin levels are high. Simultaneously, nausea and headaches along with a decrease in libido also occurs at the same time.

All this acts as a precursor to type 2 diabetes, cancer, heart disease, etc. You should also pay attention to your diet because if you load yourself with glucose derived from food that contains processed carbohydrates, you are literally knocking on the doors of hell. Not only does it reduce magnesium that is important for muscle relaxation, but it also constricts blood cells and increases the blood pressure! Look at everything insulin resistance can actually do.

I explained how you get unresponsive to something before, but it's worth mentioning again that you become insensitive towards something that occurs repeatedly. An air-hostess may find it impossible to work because she finds the harsh sound of a jet plane unbearable. But, the same air-hostess will adapt quickly and stop responding to that sound a few days later. That's how insulin resistance works.

Insulin resistance is a very common problem among many people all over the globe. It's estimated that almost 1.25 million people suffer from it in the US alone! And, don't get confused between insulin resistance and insulin sensitivity. They are not the same. In fact, they are opposite to each other.

Diet is very important if you want to deal with obesity. Most obese people struggle with belly fat. According to me, belly fat is the worst because it not only takes a long time for the body to burn the fat, but it's also more dangerous than you think. The body stores belly fat in such a way that it surrounds other organs. This visceral fat also produces fatty acids and it's released into the bloodstream. At the same time, other inflammatory hormones are also produced, further driving up insulin resistance. So, it becomes a vicious cycle again.

But, since getting rid of belly fat seems almost impossible, how do you even begin to lose the fat? Well, well, well... you can do it by practicing intermittent fasting. You can actually burn the fat around the organs by fasting. I recommend that you start today before it turns into a disease.

Sometimes, skinny people also have belly fat. They aren't obese, but their belly looks prominent. Although it doesn't look good, they aren't threatened by belly fat as much as obese people are. And that's why you should start fasting if you're obese.

Insulin resistance also worsens if you don't focus on physical activity. But. make sure that your focus is a lot more on what you eat. The point is — start fasting. It may sound difficult but you're actually doing your body a favor by not stuffing everything into your mouth all through the day.

Intermittent fasting helps you clear out your inventory before you get new stock. If you stop insulin secretion even if it's for a short while, you give your body a chance to burn all the stored fat because it will not happen in the presence of insulin. Even the levels of blood sugar become normal if you start fasting. Fat stores surrounding the midsection will burn faster and we will begin to build necessary insulin sensitivity.

The good news is that if you prepare your body to build insulin sensitivity, you are already successful in preventing most diseases. Like they say, prevention is better than cure. And the added benefit is that you heal faster. Intermittent fasting can reverse insulin resistance, so why not start today?

## Leptin Resistance

Leptin first garnered attention when Dr. Alfred met a boy who suddenly displayed signs of obesity. This happened in <u>1890</u>.

Eventually, it was declared that he had a lesion in his hypothalamus. Later, it was <u>discovered</u> that any damage to the hypothalamus resulted in obesity. Obviously, physicians realized that the hypothalamus played an important role in exaggerating obesity. By this, it was easily concluded that the hypothalamus regulated the balance of energy in the body. Also, it was now easy to understand that obesity was a result of hormonal imbalance.

But why? Why do you become obese due to the hypothalamus? Basically, the hypothalamus is responsible for regulating incoming signals that control the body's energy expenditure. It was also discovered that there were fat cells that produced a satiety factor. Whenever the fat stores grew larger in numbers, the satiety factor also increased. Now, this circulates in the blood, but once it reaches the hypothalamus, it sends signals to stop eating. In other words, it decreases the appetite and also increases metabolism. This is the body's mechanism to prevent you from becoming obese or overweight.

Also, it was discovered that the neurons present in the hypothalamus set the ideal weight, or BSW (body set weight). Any damage to this area, whether it's an injury, radiation or a tumor caused drastic obesity. The patients find it really tough to reduce weight even with a diet consisting of very few calories.

Naturally, scientists were very eager to do more research on the satiety factor. And that was none other than leptin. Leptin was discovered fairly recently in <u>1994 by Friedman.</u> Leptin's main function is to prevent cells from storing fat. To do that, it reduces hunger. If you don't have leptin, you will constantly yearn for more food. As a result, you become obese.

Consequently, scientists found rare cases of humans suffering from leptin deficiency. By treating them with leptin, they noticed drastic reversals of obesity. Obviously, the scientists were excited beyond imagination. Finally, they could solve the enigma surrounding obesity. However, they encountered a problem soon.

Sure, leptin did play a significant role in cases where obesity was prevalent, but they weren't sure about how it actually did that. Moreover, their hopes were crushed when they administered leptin to patients.

And what happened? Nothing... the patients didn't lose weight. Not that they gave up after just one study. They conducted a number of tests, but the result was the same – the participants didn't lose weight. Fact is that people with obesity do not suffer from leptin deficiency. On the contrary, they display high levels of leptin. Despite such high levels, they do not reduce weight.

How is it possible that obese people don't lose weight even with high levels of leptin when its job is to reduce hunger, you ask? Basically, if you're obese, you are resisting leptin. Leptin does work with people with normal weight. It regulates weight to a great extent. But obese people, despite having leptin, resist it and it has no effect on their weight.

So, you know now that leptin controls hunger. You'd eat a lot more if you didn't have enough leptin. And, that's why you feel hungry as soon as the levels of leptin go down. The metabolic rate also decreases consequently. Similarly, if you have a lot of leptin, you will not feel hungry. Thus, your metabolic rate increases too.

Why does this happen? It's because of the close relationship leptin shares with thyroid hormones. They are responsible for regualting development, healing, growth and metabolism in the body. As soon as you consume a meal, leptin increases and also cuts down the hunger. Or, this can happen in the midst of a meal where you're eating much more than you actually can. This is also why we find it difficult to eat more once our stomach is full.

Once leptin increases, thyroid hormones are released and it further increases the metabolism. And, this is how the body achieves a state of homeostasis or balance. As you already know, people that are leaner have low leptin levels while obese people have high levels. However, since obese people are resistant to leptin, they are unable to reduce weight.

But why does this happen? It's pretty easy to understand. Fat cells send messages to the brain by releasing leptin. They indicate that there's a lot of stored fat, which means that the individual is full and should stop eating.

In other words, the fat cells are saying that we must burn more energy and eat less. What this also means is that the fat cells produce leptin based on their size. Thus, the more obese you are, the levels of leptin are larger. Contrarily, the stored fat also decreases along with leptin when we spend some time without eating, which means that we feel hungry.

So, if the leptin levels are high, why don't people stop eating even they when are obese? The levels of leptin should signal to the brain that it's time to stop consuming food and burn more energy. Technically, it should work like that, but unfortunately leptin signals don't work properly when you're obese. Although there are high levels of leptin floating in the body, the brain becomes unresponsive and thinks that leptin levels are low! And this state is known as leptin resistance.

Remember insulin resistance due to high levels of insulin? Similarly, we develop leptin resistance when there are abnormally high levels of leptin. Although the brain does respond initially, it becomes numb or resistant to the signals over a period of time. It begins to think that the body is literally starving due to low leptin.

And when the brain stops sending messages to the body to stop eating, you don't stop eating.

At this point, the brain commits another mistake that further makes things worse for obese people. Since it thinks that we are starving, it sends signals that we should consume more food. And it also decreases the body's metabolism so that it helps us conserve a lot more energy. Due to this process, we don't burn too many calories and the body weight remains intact.

But remember I said that the thyroid hormones released concurrently with leptin help with metabolism? Yes, that's true. Then how does the brain manage to reduce metabolism despite high levels of leptin? Well, it's because the thyroid hormones don't work properly due to leptin resistance. It goes into a mode of starvation and refuses to function since the hypothalamus fails to identify high levels of leptin.

The thyroid hormones that are actually supposed to increase metabolism work in an opposite manner and lower the metabolism. The hypothalamus and thyroid hormones now think that we are starving and do everything in their power to prevent a system shut-down. Due to these fake signals, it becomes almost impossible for obese people to reduce weight. When the body itself actively refuses to lose weight, how is it even possible to become leaner? Even if you hit the gym or eat fewer calories, the body resists it.

As a result, we feel sluggish and there's a definite loss of energy. We also gain more weight because...well the brain just isn't getting it. This is why it's so hard to lose weight once we become obese. We develop leptin resistance and also become obese over time.

So, is there no hope at all? I'm already obese, and I find it difficult to shed weight, but will I ever be able to cut down my weight, you ask? YES! You can still lose weight! Because you can reset leptin resistance and turn it into leptin sensitivity!

Intermittent fasting comes in to help you out yet again! Why? Because it improves leptin resistance and makes it easier to lose weight. It also fights against inflammation and reduces triglycerides. People that are obese especially at the midsection should pay careful attention here. If you've found it impossible to reduce belly fat, it's only because your body is now resistant to leptin. This is also why we feel hungry constantly.

When you practice intermittent fasting, you'll not only reduce weight drastically but you'll also be able to shed that belly fat! Something you've been trying for years!

## Ghrelin – The hunger hormone

Ghrelin, known as the hunger hormone, sends hunger messages to the hypothalamus. It dictates when you should eat. Ever wonder why you feel so hungry when you haven't eaten anything? It's due to ghrelin. However, when you eat something and feel full, the body stops releasing ghrelin.

Ghrelin levels are high just before you eat. Conversely, they are low after you've just consumed something. This is true for those who enjoy a normal weight. However, for obese people, levels of ghrelin are lower compared to leaner people. Also, the problem is that when obese people ingest a meal, ghrelin levels go down in small quantities. Meaning, there's no reduction of hunger hormones. Or they don't feel full even after eating a meal.

If you're lean, you feel satisfied and full after a meal because the hypothalamus works perfectly and receives signals that you're done with the meal. But for obese people, the signals don't work properly. This is why we eat a lot more when we are obese.

Also, things are never easy for us when we are obese. Different myths make it literally impossible to take right decisions. For instance, people believe that dieting is as simple as counting calories. They also believe that eating a bag of chips equivalent to 100 calories is the same as eating 100 calories of green leaves! What's more alarming is that even a few physicians advocate this!

While it is true that a calorie of energy is the same no matter what, the human body refuses to agree. It's not that simple. If it was, we'd all be eating junk food and counting calories. 100 calories of say, kale, will not affect you the same way a bag of chips will! It also has something to do with the hormones produced by the body. Food react differently to the hormones.

For example, consider glucose and fructose. Glucose is present in several foods and is a natural part of our body. However, fructose is not. The human body doesn't produce fructose but it is present in processed foods. Granted that both glucose and fructose are similar due to their chemical formula, but does that make them both the same? Fructose is present in ripe fruits, but does that make any difference to the human body? No, it processes things differently.

For the human body, glucose and fructose are different. While all the tissues metabolize glucose pretty easily, only the liver can help in metabolizing fructose. But, why are we talking about all this while discussing about ghrelin? It's because glucose helps to suppress ghrelin and helps to stimulate leptin.

Coming back to fructose, it builds a lot of pressure on the liver. This results in the production of visceral fat that's really difficult to get rid of. No wonder we struggle so much to shed weight around the abdominal area, eh? Due to this pressure, the body also produces lots of waste such as uric acid that ultimately results in Gout when uric acid increases beyond limitations.

In addition, fructose is also converted into triglycerides and cholesterol that's very harmful to the body. All this gets stored as nothing but fat. Note that if you can ingest 100 calories of glucose, the body stores very few calories as fat. In fact, it's less than 1 calorie. But the body stores more than 30 calories as fat when you ingest 100 calories of fructose.

Since glucose has the ability to suppress ghrelin, it indirectly suppresses the appetite. Unfortunately, fructose leads to high levels of ghrelin compared to glucose. So, what happens then? Yes, you guessed that right – it makes you hungrier than ever. Fructose slyly interferes with the signals the brain sends and it makes you overeat.

Fructose actually leads to insulin resistance due to all the overeating too. It doesn't satisfy you in the same way glucose does. Yes, glucose and fructose may have the same number of calories but the body processes it very differently. Now you know that a calorie of one type of food is not equivalent to a calorie of another type of food.

Note that I'm only referring to fructose derived from commercially processed foods. It's not the same as fructose derived from ripe fruits. It's because fruits make you chew and they also contain loads of water and fiber that work diligently to avoid the effects of fructose.

So what does this tell you? The moral of the story is that you must reduce processed food. Especially the ones that contain lots of processed sugar. Get into the habit of reading labels, and stay away from foods containing fructose. By replacing junk food with foods containing protein and good fat, you will be able to reduce ghrelin and in turn feel less hungry.

Reduce carbs as much as possible. This is also why low-carb diets are popular and actually work. It reduces your appetite and you begin eating fewer calories since insulin, leptin and ghrelin all work together to help you shed weight.

Most importantly, don't worry too much about counting calories. Like explained already, it's a futile exercise. It's not necessary to lose weight just because you're eating fewer calories. Think more becoming healthier and you will shine!

All this is awesome, but what's the connection between ghrelin and intermittent fasting, you ask? Well, IF improves the benefits of ghrelin. Whenever ghrelin is released, we immediately consume something, and it decreases ghrelin levels. However, we are ultimately missing out on lots of things including the production of HGH that will be discussed in the next chapter.

Just when the body decides to produce HGH and improve growth, repair and other important functions, we immediately eat something and reduce ghrelin and HGH. Ghrelin indirectly increases HGH. Thus, by decreasing ghrelin, we are constantly reducing the chances of tissue repair, growth and healing.

To increase ghrelin and HGH, ensure that you work out after fasting for several hours. If you're obese, ghrelin levels are low, and HGH isn't released properly. Thus, it's your responsibility to make sure that you practice IF so that the hormones start functioning properly.

What if you're working out in the morning? Don't want to miss out on breakfast because it's supposedly the most critical meal of the day? Ha, that's a joke. Breakfast actually cuts down on ghrelin levels as soon as you start the day. No matter how much they tell you to stuff yourself as soon as you wake up, the truth remains that breakfast isn't actually helping you. Doughnuts, pastries, muffins, chocolate chips, cookies and other sugary stuff that you eat for breakfast literally smashes your chances of becoming leaner.

Thus, remember and think of ghrelin when you're hungry next time. You'll hear your stomach growling but treat that as music because it only means that you're on the path to becoming fitter and leaner.

# Chapter 8
# Connection between the growth hormone and insulin

Also known as HGH, the human growth hormone is created by a gland known as the pituitary gland. It is a hormone that's released in small bursts. HGH levels often rise after you exercise or sleep. It also occurs when you experience something traumatic.

Due to its relationship with insulin, it so happens that the levels of HGH is high during nighttime compared to daytime. As you progress in age from your childhood and hit puberty, the levels of HGH also rise; however, it starts declining once you reach middle age.

But how is the HGH connected to insulin, you ask? Well, you already know the hormone insulin rises whenever you ingest food. Insulin, as I've mentioned before, helps you process sugar and transport it into the bloodstream. Whenever you need energy to do pretty much anything, insulin does its job.

When you are sensitive to insulin, the food you consume is also used in an efficient manner. In addition, the more sensitivity you display, the more HGH is produced. Thus, it's simple to understand that as the levels of insulin increase, HGH decreases. It's important to note here that the pituitary glands release HGH only when there's no presence of insulin in the bloodstream. But when does your body reach a state where there's less insulin produced? Yes, it happens either when you're sleeping or when you're fasting.

Wonder why that happens? It's because when you're in a rested state or sleeping, there's no glucose entering your bloodstream due to a meal you have consumed recently. Thus, there's no insulin released. At the same time, HGH is released since there isn't a lot of insulin. The body displays maximum sensitivity to insulin when you're fasting. The same thing happens when you're sleeping.

This tells you what exactly you need to do if you want to reduce weight. However, most of us do the opposite. Remember I said that insulin is released whenever you consume food? Thus, the more you eat, the more insulin is released. Talk about ingesting 6 small meals every day. Sure, you're only eating small amounts, but insulin will be released nonetheless.

Let's imagine someone's constantly yelling in your ears. If it happens frequently, you become immune to it and even start ignoring it. Same thing with medications. If you consume the same drug constantly, your body will become resistant to it. Similarly, if you have the habit of stuffing food into your mouth frequently, insulin levels increase proportionally. And what happens then? Your body becomes resistant to it. Or unresponsive.

Based on a research conducted by the American College of Cardiology, HGH increased by over 1300% for women when they fasted! It's even better for men with over 2000%! This tells you why fasting is simply the best way to not only reduce weight but also improve your fitness and lifestyle.

Also known as the fitness hormone, HGH actually promotes muscles and increases fat loss at a rapid pace. So, if you're picturing yourself as a starved person due to intermittent fasting, think again! You not only lose weight, but the bonus is that you become lean.

For athletes, intermittent fasting is a boon in disguise. Since HGH improves the way the body heals itself and also repairs tissues at a faster rate, athletes can improve their performance. When combined with training, HGH plays a key role in promoting many important elements in the body.

Instead of relying on supplements that work only temporarily, intermittent fasting can actually change your life. Even if you're worried about losing weight for cosmetic reasons, remember that fasting can actually slow down the aging process. The best part is that HGH also works similarly. It burns fat and ensures that the process of aging occurs slowly.

This is also why artificial injections of HGH are in demand. The only problem is that they are synthetic. It makes no sense to rely on something artificial. Therefore, it's best on do something naturally like IF and gain utmost benefits from it.

# Chapter 9
# Myths about fasting

When I told a friend of mine that I was going to fast for a day, she was so terrified that her eyes bulged out of her sockets. Many people believe that fasting for 24-48 hours can actually kill you. There's no dearth of misinformation out there, but there are innumerable theories on fasting and most of them point towards a myth that fasting can be fatal. Here are a few myths about fasting your friends and well-wishers may tell you. Although they believe that they are helping you, you now know that the reality is different.

## Myth 1 – You must eat frequently

Boy, this myth is just too rampant. Often perpetuated by companies selling packaged food, many people actually believe that eating frequently is beneficial. But why? Well, they think that it increases the metabolic rate that in turn helps you lose weight.

Fact is that while the metabolic rate does increase when you eat frequently, there's not much of a difference. It's like counting pennies while ignoring $100 bills. The metabolic rate doesn't increase so much that you get rid of the fat. Instead, what happens is that the body begins to store all that extra food as fat…and then…viola – you simply put on weight.

If you believe in this myth and actually eat six times a day to increase the metabolic rate, you're not going to lose weight because you're going to need a lot more time to shed all that extra fat that gets stored.

## Myth 2 – Fasting makes you lose your muscles

So, what this myth means is that if you fast for a while, the body begins to burn your own muscles, and you're ultimately going to have no muscles or protein. Seriously, this myth's the funniest of all. It's hilarious because it has absolutely no logic. Nada. None.

Let's imagine for a second that this myth is true. But how would you explain how humans survived when there was no food at all? What about the days when humans had to hunt? Or what about those days when men and women including children had to go for days without food when their countries were engaged in wars? They would all be dead by now. And the human race would have vanished, right?

If the human body indeed started burning or eating its own muscles due to a fast, you would fall sick right after your first fast. Nobody would fast at all because it would simply mean certain death. And the human body wouldn't store fat to burn it as energy later if it planned to burn muscles instead.

Sure, starvation does break muscles down, but you'd have to be severely starved for that. That would mean that you aren't eating or drinking anything for months together. When the body realizes that there's absolutely no fat in the system it burns muscles, but you'd have to starve for days and even months at a stretch to come to that point.

Let me reiterate here again that fasting and starving isn't the same thing. There's no control over starving while fasting is completely in your hands. You're the driver in the seat, and you know exactly what you're doing, so do not get confused between the two.

## Myth 3 – Brain cells die when you fast

This is, by far, the worst I've seen. Some people actually believe that brain cells stop functioning due to fasting because there's a depletion in glucose. Say what? Yes, they think that fasting forces the brain to shut down just because there's no glucose.

This misconception is absolutely incorrect. Glucose decreases or depletes from the human body just within 24 hours. It's a fact. So, if the myth were to be true, we'd all be brain-dead just within 24 hours. People who have fasted to detoxify their bodies even centuries ago would be brain-dead after just a day of fasting.

What about the homeless that survive for days without food? They become weak, of course, but do they lose their marbles? Nope. The truth is that the human brain uses ketones while conserving protein during starvation. Glucose is necessary, sure, but it's not the ultimate source for survival. Once glucose depletes from the human body, it uses long-term stores or fat, as you already know, and that's how you lose weight. It's the very concept of Intermittent Fasting.

## Myth 4 – You will face extreme hunger when fasting

Most studies on fasting suggest that although the subjects felt hungry during the first two days, their bodies adjusted pretty nicely to the routine. Extreme cases show that a few individuals have fasted for more than 100 days and survived on nothing but water, tea and coffee.

Yes, you will be hungry at the very beginning. However, as the day progresses, the feeling of hunger diminishes. It will be uncomfortable, but it's bearable. Most importantly, hunger pangs come and go in short waves – something very similar to the feeling you get after quitting cigarettes. As long as you keep yourself busy and stop thinking about the hunger, you'll be okay.

## Myth 5 – Fasting decreases metabolism

Yet another myth about fasting is that it dramatically reduces basal metabolism, ultimately becoming fatal for the person who's fasting. Like other myths, this one's not true either because although the metabolism decreases a bit when you restrict calories, the body switches to burning all the stored fat when you start fasting.

## Myth 6 – Fasting leads to overeating

According to this myth, this is how it goes: You fast on day 1 and eat more on day 2. Actually, there is some truth to it where you do eat a bit more on day 2. However, it's nowhere close to overeating. Let me explain. Studies reflect an increase in calories on the second day, but it's minimal.

For instance, let's imagine you fasted on day 1 and consumed 2300 calories on day 2 instead of ingesting your regular 2000 calories. However, note that that you now ingested only 2300 for two days rather than 4000. That's a large difference. Thus, although you may eat a little more on the days you don't fast, it certainly doesn't add up. Plus, appetite decreases after you begin fasting frequently, so it's a win-win!

# Chapter 10
# Common questions on fasting

Naturally, you're going to have a lot of questions before beginning your fast, so this section is dedicated to answering all the questions you'll probably have. Fasting refers to a period where you consume absolutely nothing, including water and food; however, you'll be drinking lots of water during your fast to avoid dehydration.

First of all, fasting doesn't come with a fixed time duration. You can fast for a day or even 30 days, depending on your goal. However, IF fasting is a stage where you allow your body to feast and fast intermittently. Thus, it makes sense to stick to shorter time frames and see how your body adjusts to it.

While some people swear by the 16:8 fast where they eat only during an 8-hour window, others prefer fasting for 24 hours and eating normally the next day. Whatever you do, make sure your body adjusts to it rather than forcing it because you'll simply quit after a while.

So, you know how the 16:8 fast works. You fast for 16 hours, and eat only during the remaining 8 hours. A 24-hour fast means you simply can't consume anything for one full day. Thus, if you eat dinner today at 8 pm, you cannot eat anything until 8 pm the next day. Some people extend this to 36 hours. And, this means that if you eat dinner at 8 pm tonight on a Wednesday, you cannot eat anything until 8 am on Friday.

Most of these protocols work; however, fasting for long periods of time (at least 24 hours) regularly will make a great difference. This is because your insulin levels decrease to a great extent and losing weight becomes super easy. Your blood sugar also decreases. But, if you feel extremely nauseous, you might have to stop and determine what's actually wrong.

## What can I consume while fasting?

Generally, while fasting, you cannot consume any solid food. However, liquid food is allowed as long as it doesn't contain any sugar. Not even tender coconuts because it contains sugar. Or even sugarcane juice for that matter. If you love drinking lemon water with honey as soon as you wake up, you must skip adding honey during fasting days because although honey is natural, it contains sugar.

You goal must be to drink as much water as possible when fasting. Honestly, that's the trick behind staying sane when you aren't eating anything. And water clears your skin, hydrates you, and also makes you lose weight simultaneously. What's not to love?!

Start off by drinking at least a liter of water every day. As you go on, increase the water intake until you drink about 3 liters every day. You can also add lemon or vinegar to add a little flavor. Vinegar actually aids with your blood sugar. But adding flavors may not work for many. For instance, I feel nauseous when I drink lemon water on an empty stomach, so I drink only plain water.

You can also add ginger or cucumber slices to your water. But just stay away from artificial flavors like Tang because they contain loads of sugar. Fruit juices are strictly not allowed, because, yes...they contain sugar.

Coming to other beverages, you can drink as much coffee as you want. But remember to not add sugar of any kind whether it's natural or artificial. No brown sugar either. Adding a little amount of milk or cream is okay, but since they contain sugar, remember not to overdo it. You don't want to fast the entire day and waste it all just because you added a lot of milk now, do you?

If hunger pangs are too much, you can drink a bit of bone broth, but make sure you prepare it at home instead of purchasing commercial ones. Also don't add bouillon cubes because they contain sugar and other artificial elements.

Even vegetable broth is an excellent addition when you're fasting. You can add salt to your broths since you're not consuming salt at all.

## How to break the fast?

Say you're going for a 24-hour fast. That means that if you're going to have breakfast at 8 am today, you can only eat at 8 am the next day. To break the fast, drink some water and then eat a little of whatever you've planned. Don't go all out and stuff yourself or it will make you uncomfortable.

## Is it possible to exercise when fasting?

Absolutely! In fact, it's recommended that you exercise when fasting because your body burns all the extra fat as soon as possible. It's like the icing on the cake. Any type of exercise is okay. Many people believe that you can't exercise because there's no energy when you aren't eating but that's not true because the liver is responsible for supplying energy through gluconeogenesis. The human body is such an amazing machine that the muscles utilize fatty acids to derive energy.

Fasting also makes you alert and kicks off your adrenaline. In fact, there's an increase in growth hormones that work wonderfully when you exercise. An increase in muscle growth also explains why some people rely on exercising while fasting to tone their bodies.

## How to ignore hunger when fasting?

This is a common question, and one that scares the bejesus out of people everywhere. But, it's not that bad. Just ask someone who has tried IF. They will tell you that it's quite easy once you get the hang of it. You will not be hungry at all for the first 3-4 hours. In fact, many people don't feel hungry for the first 8 hours. Of course, you will feel a few hunger pangs after that. To counter that, sip water slowly until the hunger subsides and you'll be okay.

As mentioned above, you can also drink vegetable or bone broth to gain some nutrients and stave off your hunger for a while. If you've planned a 24-hour fast, you won't even realize how fast the time flies because you'll also count the number of hours you've slept. A 36-hour fast may be difficult, especially if you're a beginner. Thus, it's recommended that you start off with a 16:8 fast and then proceed to 24-hour fasts.

Hunger actually comes in waves. As soon as you feel hungry, distract yourself and you'll notice that you won't feel hungry after five minutes! Do not tell yourself that you're overwhelmed. Instead, convince yourself that you can do it. After all, it all depends on your mindset.

## Why do I get headaches when fasting?

Many people experience slight headaches during fasting. This is more common than you believe and is caused due to a low salt consumption. When the body transitions from a high-salt diet to literally zero salt, headaches persist. However, headaches fade away once you continue fasting. If anything, keep sipping on water with a pinch of salt to make the headaches go away.

## How do I avoid cramps during fasting?

You could get cramps if you're dehydrated. Thus, drink more water. Another reason could be that you're experiencing a depletion in magnesium that can be corrected by consuming a magnesium supplement or soaking your feet in water mixed with magnesium salts. Epsom salts – as they are commonly known – are available in all drug stores.

## Why do I experience fatigue when fasting?

Actually, fasting makes you active due to the adrenaline. Your basal metabolism also hikes up, which means that you're going to be more active. The tiredness you feel could be hunger, or it could be due to salt depletion. However, if you constantly feel extremely tired and are unable to do pretty much anything you must consult a physician because it's not something that's occurring due to fasting alone.

## Why do I get dizzy during a fast?

Some people experience mild dizziness when they fast. This is common, but this is also due to a lack of salt. Adding a little salt to water or broth may help. Another reason could be dehydration, which means that you should never forget to replenish your body with lots of water whenever possible.

## Will I experience memory loss when fasting?

Hell, no! Not only will you not experience memory loss, but you will be more focused and alert when fasting! Studies on fasting have proven that your cognitive ability increases when you're fasting. This <u>study</u> shows that fasting improved mental flexibility to a great extent.

## Why can't I sleep while fasting?

This is an issue I faced when I was fasting. You might find it difficult to sleep, especially if you've planned your fast in such a way that you can't have dinner. However, this occurs only during your initial days where hunger pangs make you toss and turn in your bed. This is natural and there's nothing alarming about it. But remember that the body adjusts quickly and you'll not experience the same if you keep up with it for at least a fortnight.

## Why do I experience acidity when fasting?

Although acidity doesn't have anything to do with fasting, it can occur due to what you eat when you're not fasting. If you're eating foods that can cause acidity, it could explain why you're experiencing acidity on a regular basis. Also, overeating during your eating window could also be the reason why you feel acidity. The best way to avoid this is to sleep at least an hour after you've finished eating. Most people experience acidity when they sleep right after a huge meal.

## Why am I experiencing issues in the bathroom?

Many people feel constipated when they fast. But this is not due to fasting. In fact, it's due to the food you eat when you're fasting. Eating foods with a lot of fiber and then fasting immediately after can result in constipation. But this can be rectified by drinking lots of water. Generally, your body adjusts to all this and the problems fade away after a while, but if the problem persists you can consider using any of the many laxatives available.

## Can I take my regular medications while fasting?

It depends on the type of medications you're using. While some medications react differently if you take it on an empty stomach, others may have no effect at all. Thus, the best way to find a solution is to consult your physician.

## What about people with diabetes?

It's difficult for people with diabetes to indulge in a fast due to the medications they consume and also because of the blood sugar that decreases when fasting. Although fasting is very beneficial for people suffering from diabetes, it's essential that you do it only if you have someone to monitor you closely.

Do not – I repeat – do not fast if you're alone and there's nobody to take care of you. Fasting when you have diabetes can make your blood sugars plummet to such a level that it can be fatal. Before you know it, it becomes a dangerous situation. Losing weight is necessary when you have diabetes, but it must be done under careful supervision.

## How much can I expect to lose?

Well, it totally depends. Not only on what you eat during your eating window, but also on the type of fast you're doing. For instance, your friend fasting every alternate day may have better luck than you who's depending on the 16:8 fast. It's also possible that you lose weight faster even if you're on the 16:8 diet because we are all different.

To make sure that you complete your fast without any hindrance, ensure that you don't discuss it with anybody. This is because many people think that fasting can be fatal, and constant discouragement can be detrimental to your goals.

Coming back to the amount of weight you can lose, remember that you will hit a plateau where you stop losing weight. This is because your metabolism decreases and your body forces you to stop losing weight. At this point of time, you'll need to make some changes. For example, if you're fasting only for 24 hours, try extending it to 36 hours and repeat it until you lose weight. By doing this, you'll also reduce your BSW (Body set weight) and ensure that all the lost weight doesn't come back.

Obese people that have gained weight slowly over the years will find it particularly hard to lose weight. This is because the body has adjusted itself to the weight gain. This is why you must persist and continue fasting until you shed all the extra weight.

## Can you give me a few tips to successfully finish my fast?

1. Make up your mind – Fasting is all about your mindset. If you think that you can't do it, you will not be able to do it. But if you convince yourself that it's easy, you will do much better. Remember that your health will also improve, so it's not only about losing weight.

2. Drink as much water as possible. It's literally your lifeline because you're not going to feel very good if you stay away

from both food and water. Dehydration is a pain and you must avoid it at all costs.

3. Try to exercise – Exercising while fasting works wonderfully. If you're too tired, a few basic exercises like stretching will also help.

4. Distract yourself – Hunger pangs are common if you're a beginner. But the best way to continue with your fast is to distract yourself. Before you know it, your fasting window would have passed by and you won't even notice it.

5. Try to forget the time period – Let's imagine you eat at 9 pm tonight. If you're doing a 24-hour fast, you can only eat the next day at 9 pm. If you constantly think about the time and wait for your eating time-frame, you're never going to be able to finish your fast. You're actually driving yourself crazy by constantly thinking about when you can eat. On the contrary, if you forget about it, you'll do much better. So, stop doing it and make it easier for yourself.

6. Give yourself a fighting chance – Give your body a fighting chance by surviving on as many liquids as possible. Water is a given, yes, but tea, coffee and even chia seeds can help you get rid of the hunger. <u>Chia seeds are full of fiber</u>. 2 tbsp contain about 10 grams of fiber. Although it's solid food, it won't make a difference to your fasting routine.

7. Stop overeating – I cannot stress this enough. Overeating just after a fast can be harmful. Not only will you suffer from heartburn, but your efforts will also go for a toss.

8. Focus on a nutritious diet on non-fasting days – Eating leafy greens and healthy salads on non-fasting days will improve your chances of losing weight.

9. Give yourself some time – In the beginning, you may be discouraged. You may also give up. But, like everything else, fasting requires determination. Give your body ample time to adjust to this new routine, and once it does, you'll not face any issues.

10. Feast when it's required – Like I said, you need to feast at times. Marriages, birthdays and parties are meant to be enjoyed. Don't be that woman who walks into a party announcing that you're fasting!

# Chapter 11
# What are the benefits of intermittent fasting

Apart from weight loss, Intermittent Fasting helps to fight against several diseases. Here are a few diseases you can either prevent or cure if you practice intermittent fasting.

## 1. Type 2 Diabetes

### What is type 2 diabetes?

Diabetes is a condition that forces the levels of blood sugar to spike up. Type 2 diabetes, in particular, is a disease that becomes worse if it's not treated. In general, the pancreas produces insulin. Due to Type 2 diabetes, the pancreas either does not produce the required insulin or the cells in the body display no reaction to insulin.

Insulin controls glucose levels in the blood. Since insulin levels are low or almost nonexistent when a patient is suffering from Type 2 diabetes, the glucose remains in the blood and is not used by the body as fuel or energy. When this happens, the body fights back and tries hard to decrease glucose levels.

Those suffering from Type 2 Diabetes generally feel thirsty, nauseous, dizzy and experience too much fatigue. They also pass a lot of urine compared to others. Another typical symptom is drastic weight loss coupled with a decrease in muscle bulk.

Basically, type 2 diabetes is much more rampant compared to type 1 diabetes. It also occurs generally due to obesity. Physicians treat patients through a combination of lifestyle changes and medications that make the blood sugar levels normal. And, talking of lifestyle changes, the patients are asked to indulge in different diets but the ultimate goal is to avoid sugar and carbs.

Intermittent Fasting seems like a suitable candidate to manage sugar levels. Many scientists have put this to test. One particular study in Canada tried IF on three subjects battling with diabetes. All the three individuals were relying on insulin to tackle diabetes. Additionally, they also had high cholesterol and blood pressure.

Diabetes is a disease that almost has no cure. It's pretty difficult for patients considering that they are stuck in a vicious cycle. Now, you know that insulin makes you put on weight. And it's important to reduce weight if you have diabetes. However, since the patients need to take insulin to counter diabetes, they find it impossible to lose weight no matter what.

But, here, the goal wasn't to reduce weight. The focus was on fighting diabetes. So, coming back to the study, all the three subjects were informed on how diabetes could affect them and how diet could help manage it. While two of the three men fasted for 24 hours on alternate days, the third subject took up a 3-day fast every week. They were allowed to drink coffee, water and tea. In addition, they also ate low-calorie meals at evenings.

What was amazing was that while two participants stopped taking insulin after 1 month since the trial, one participant stopped insulin within a mere five days! Two of the three men stopped with all the drugs they were previously subjected to while the third man could stop consuming three out of the four drugs he was using to overcome diabetes.

The experiment lasted for ten months, and the subjects noticed an immense improvement in their weight. Apparently, they didn't encounter any difficulties while fasting either. What was amazing was that while their blood glucose levels lowered significantly, they also lost weight. Losing weight is an afterthought in this experiment. Instead, we should focus on how IF helped them overcome diabetes – a disease that almost has no cure!

At the end of the trial, the scientists were convinced that IF helps with diabetes, but since they had experimented only on three participants, they concluded that it warranted more research. They also stated that 24-hour fasts could help people with diabetes significantly.

Another <u>study</u> published in a well-known journal named Autophagy tested IF on mice. They found that Intermittent Fasting helped to preserve the beta cells of the mice that were initially afflicted with diabetes induced by obesity. Type 2 diabetes is a combination of insulin resistance and a reduction of beta cells. Ultimately, the researchers found that IF helped to preserve those beta cells.

Although the research is promising, it's important to note that mice and humans are not the same. The human body is complex and certainly differs from that of mice, but the fact that IF helped mice afflicted with diabetes is promising nonetheless.

Let's take a look at another study that was published in none other than the World Journal of Diabetes. The aim of the study was to determine the effects of IF on adults afflicted with type 2 diabetes.

The scientists conducted tests on ten individuals. The blood glucose levels of all the subjects were tested throughout the study to see if IF brought any significant changes. Finally, they also collected blood samples at the end of every study phase.

Note that all the ten subjects were obese and were consuming metformin – a medication used to reduce blood sugar levels. At the end of the study, the scientists noted that the subjects lost weight considerably. They also displayed a reduction in blood glucose levels. Thus, the researchers concluded that IF was a safe and effective way to counter diabetes. Although the number of participants were less, these studies give a lot of hope for patients that are hopeless when it comes to diabetes.

## 2. Heart Health

Unfortunately, you cannot find many studies of how IF improves heart health. But what we have seen so far is promising. Scientists are not really sure why, but apparently IF does improve heart health and also reduces risk factors that are related to the heart.

Some studies indicate that practicing IF regularly can help the heart in many ways. This is because of the way the human body metabolizes sugar and cholesterol. It also decreases the bad cholesterol or low-density lipoprotein present in the body.

IF may sound like a fabulous dieting craze to many, but the truth is that we need more research to help many people suffering from various diseases. In one <u>study</u> conducted by scientists at Intermountain Healthcare, they found that patients that indulged in IF regularly had a higher chance of living longer than people that didn't practice IF.

They also found that individuals that frequently fasted had a lesser risk of heart failure. The scientists presented their findings where more than 2000 patients were asked a series of questions to determine how IF helped change their lives. What's more interesting is that the scientists went back to those patients almost 5 years later. Interestingly, they concluded that the patients that practiced IF had a higher chance of survival compared to those that didn't follow IF.

According to this particular <u>journal</u>, a lot of improvements were shown also in mice due to IF. They also found significant weight loss in humans. The researchers found significant reduction in leptin and insulin levels along with body fat. While the ketone levels had increased, the blood pressure and heart rate had decreased.

A few more studies on the effect of IF related to heart diseases will further strengthen our belief that IF not only helps you reduce weight, but it can also reduce risks related to the heart.

## 3. Alzheimer's disease

Alzheimer's is a disease where the brain cells die and eventually cause an impairment in your cognitive abilities. It is a neurological disorder and although you see mild symptoms at first, it worsens in the later stages.

According to this study, scientists tested the effects of Intermittent Fasting on mice. Their findings state that the cortisol levels that had increased abnormally due to Alzheimer's was reduced due to IF. Additionally, their study indicated that IF improved liver damage and reduced memory loss.

Until now, we haven't seen any studies conducted on humans, but since there's so much evidence of IF doing wonders on animals, we can hope that it helps us mortals too.

# Conclusion

Intermittent Fasting can be hard. Yes, it sure is. And it will be harder if you don't convince yourself that it's only for your well-being. The truth is that nothing comes easy in life. And, obesity is super hard to get rid of once you pack all those pounds.

But don't lose heart. That's the most important thing. You must remember that it only becomes better. It becomes easy from the second week. Your stomach will growl. You'll even hear churning noises. But it's your responsibility to ignore that. You may feel a bit weak during week 1, but that too shall pass.

In fact, you only become more active and alert after a while. Apart from losing unwanted fat, you'll even become fitter and ready to take on the world. And since I am writing this book while practicing intermittent fasting, it's proof that you can do anything if you only put your mind to it.

I hope you seriously practice IF because it's the only way to reduce your weight. As a woman, you'll regain confidence and even fit into the smallest of dresses! I've explained already that IF is the same for both men and women, so don't let poorly-researched articles bother you. Most importantly, it can save your life, so go for it girl!

If you've enjoyed reading this book, subscribe* to my mailing list for exclusive content and sneak peeks of my future books.

Visit the link below:

http://eepurl.com/gJnw1X

**OR**

Use the QR Code:

(*Must be 13 years or older to subscribe)

www.ingramcontent.com/pod-product-compliance
Lightning Source LLC
Chambersburg PA
CBHW051215250726
48655CB00006B/2425